James
and
Awesome Autism

PAGE PUBLISHING, INC.
New York, NY

First originally published by Page Publishing, Inc. 2018

ISBN 978-1-64350-181-9 (Paperback)
ISBN 978-1-64350-183-3 (Digital)

Printed in the United States of America

James
and
Awesome Autism

Carmela Fazio-Florio

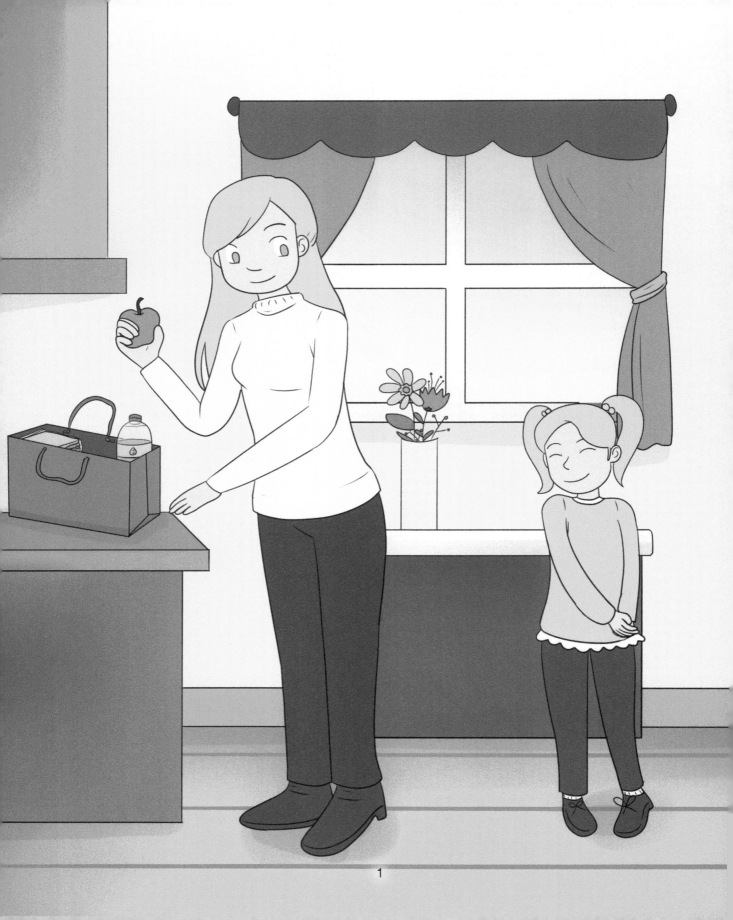

It was a beautiful, sunny day in New York City. Lilly woke up early Saturday morning.

"Mommy," said Lilly, "can we go to the park, please?"

"Okay," said Lilly's mom, Jennifer. "We will go in a bit." Lilly was so excited to spend some time with her mom. After all, it was a long week in the first grade. Lilly packed a lunch bag with all her favorite snacks and drinks: Goldfish, granola bars, and fruit punch, to name a few.

When Lilly got to the park, there were so many fun things to do there. She saw a slide and some swings.

"Mommy," said Lilly, "I want to go play on the swings."

"Okay, hon," Jennifer replied.

Jennifer sat on the bench, reading her book while watching Lilly play with the other children. Lilly went from the swings, to the slide, and then back to the swings again. Lilly was having so much fun! It was such a beautiful October day in fall!

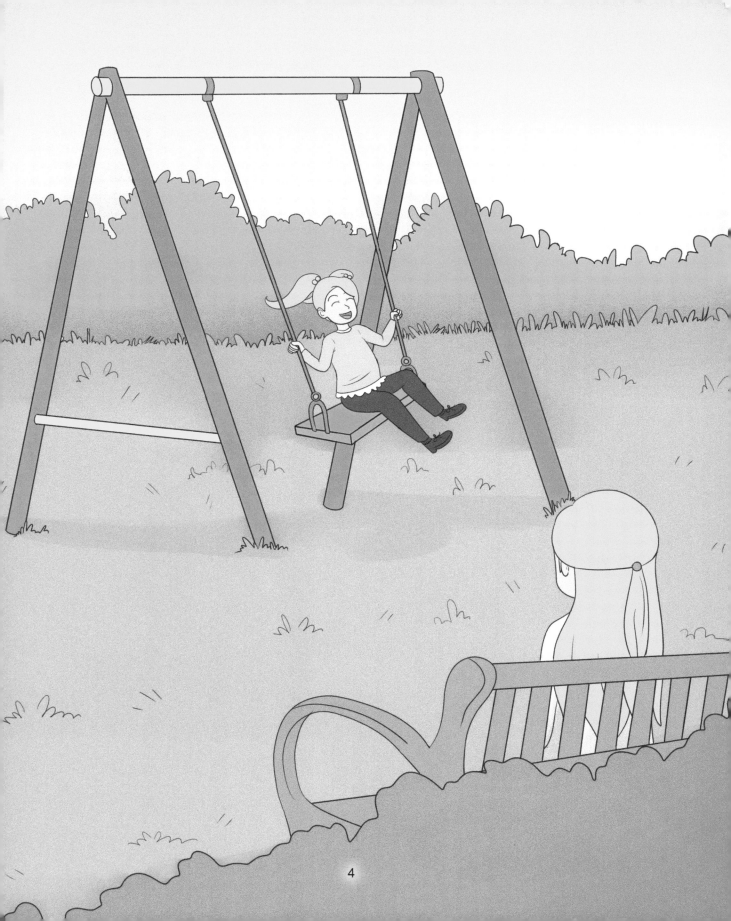

Jennifer spotted a little boy playing by himself in the corner. Lilly went up to the little boy and said, "Hi there! Want to play on the swings?" There was no response. Once again, Lilly asked, "Hi, do you want to come play?" Still there was no response.

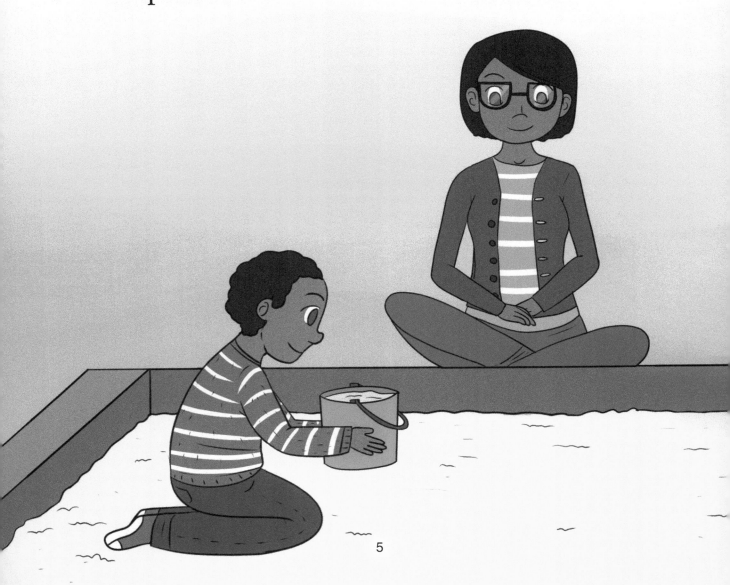

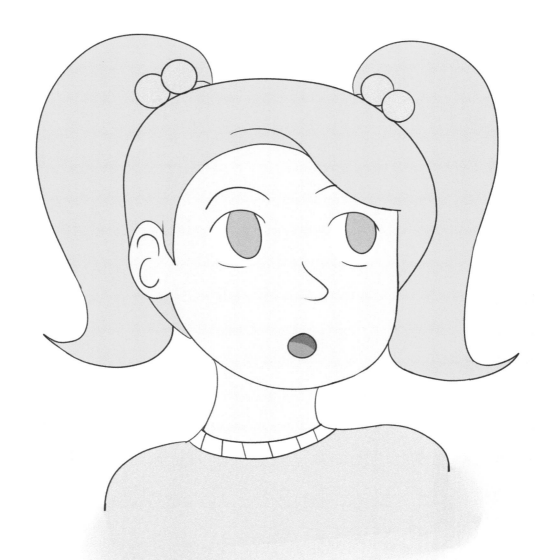

He was not even looking at her, almost ignoring her. Then he began to throw sand up in the air, and some got in Lilly's face. Lilly felt so sad, her eyes filled up with tears, and she began to cry. She ran to her mom.

"Mommy, Mommy," she cried. "Why is that boy being so mean to me? First he was ignoring me, and now he's throwing sand."

Jennifer looked over at the little boy. She saw his mother go over to him to tell him to stop throwing sand, but he continued. He dropped to the floor and started crying uncontrollably. He started to scream, cover his ears, and rock back and forth. Everyone at the park was staring.

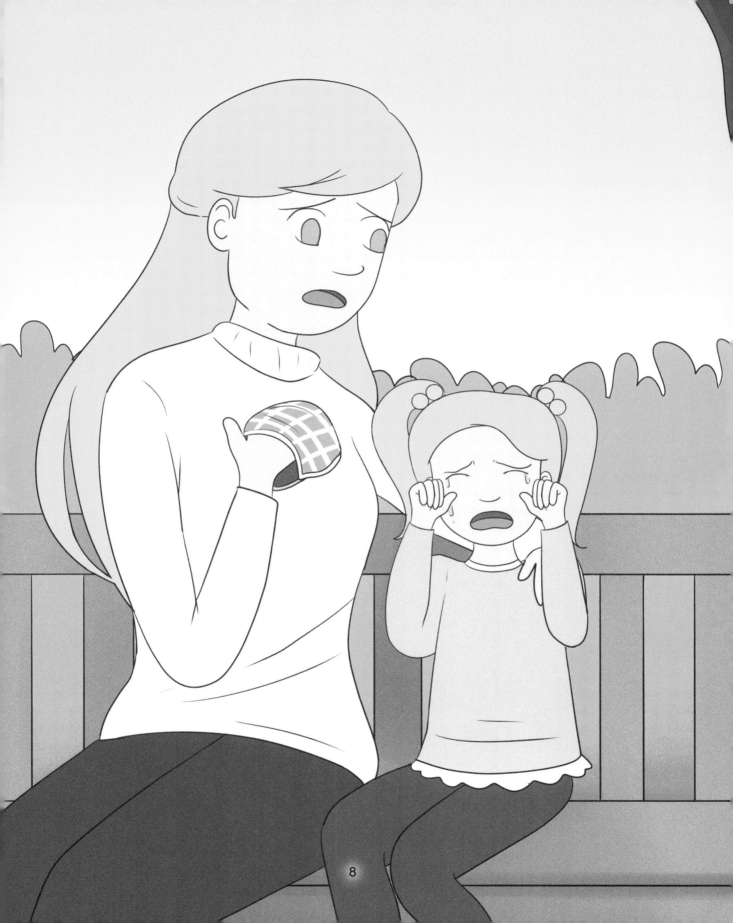

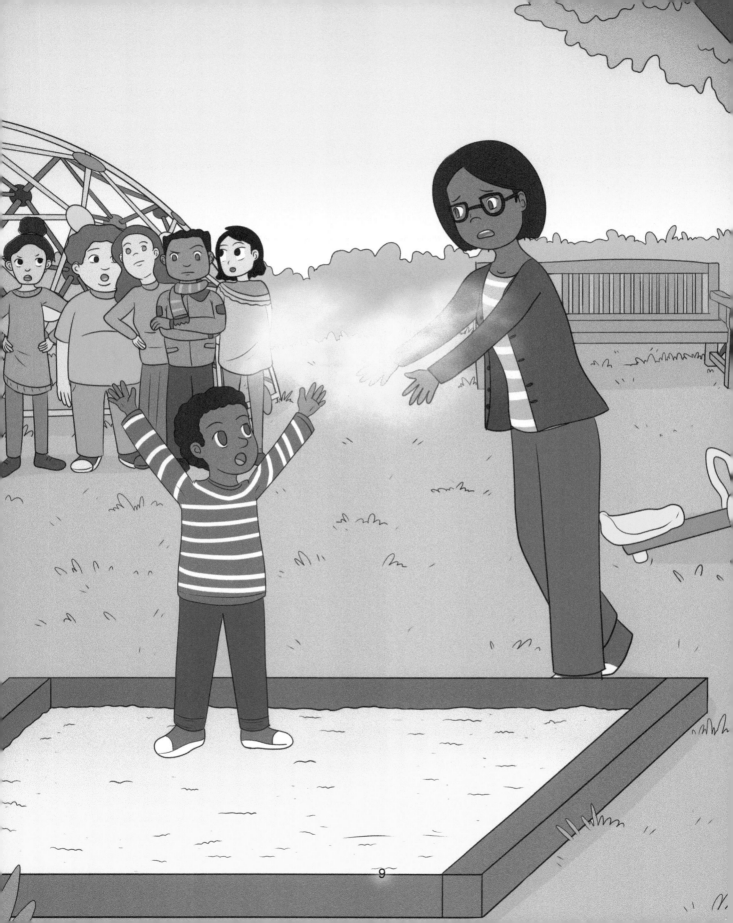

People were making comments.

"Get some control over that kid!" one old man yelled.

"He's scaring my daughter!" moaned another.

"Something's wrong, Mommy," Lilly said.

"What's going on?" Jennifer walked over and offered help to the other mother. She placed her hand on her shoulder and, with a friendly smile, said, "Is there anything I can do to help?"

The woman sadly looked at Jennifer and said, "My son James has autism. He is having a meltdown because I wanted him to stop throwing the sand."

"Oh, I see," Jennifer said. "Would James like a snack? We have some Goldfish, Oreo cookies, and chips in our lunch bag."

"James loves Goldfish!" his mom, Angela, exclaimed.

"Great," Jennifer said, "I'll go get some!" Jennifer came back with Lilly and a bag of Goldfish. Lilly held out her hand.

"Here," said Lilly as she held out the bag to James with a big smile. James took the Goldfish out of Lilly's hand. He began to eat them, and slowly he started to calm down.

"Thank you, sweetie," said Angela.

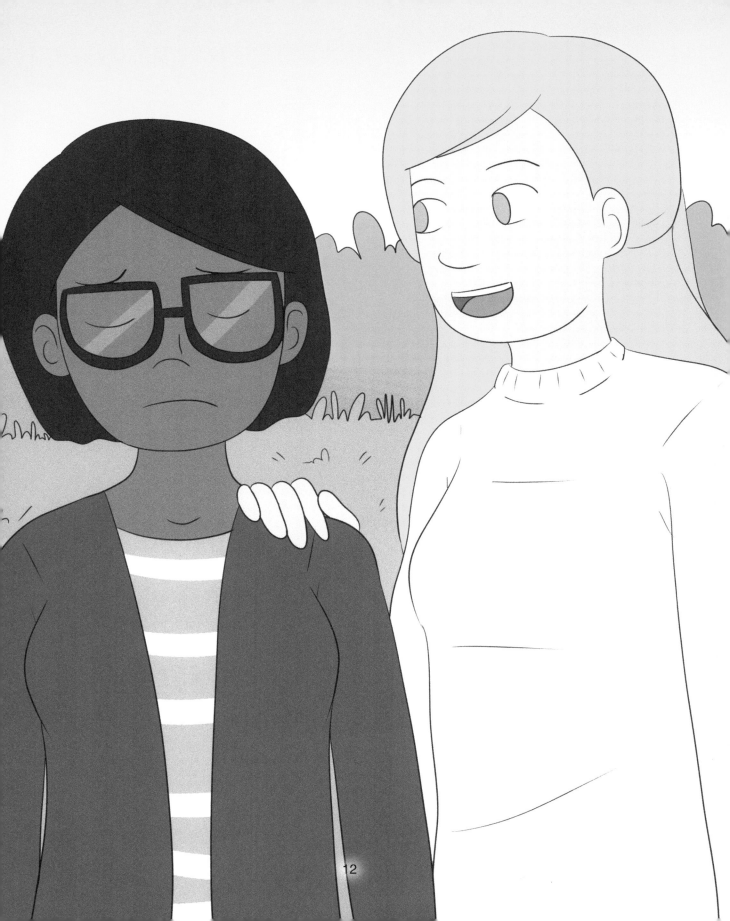

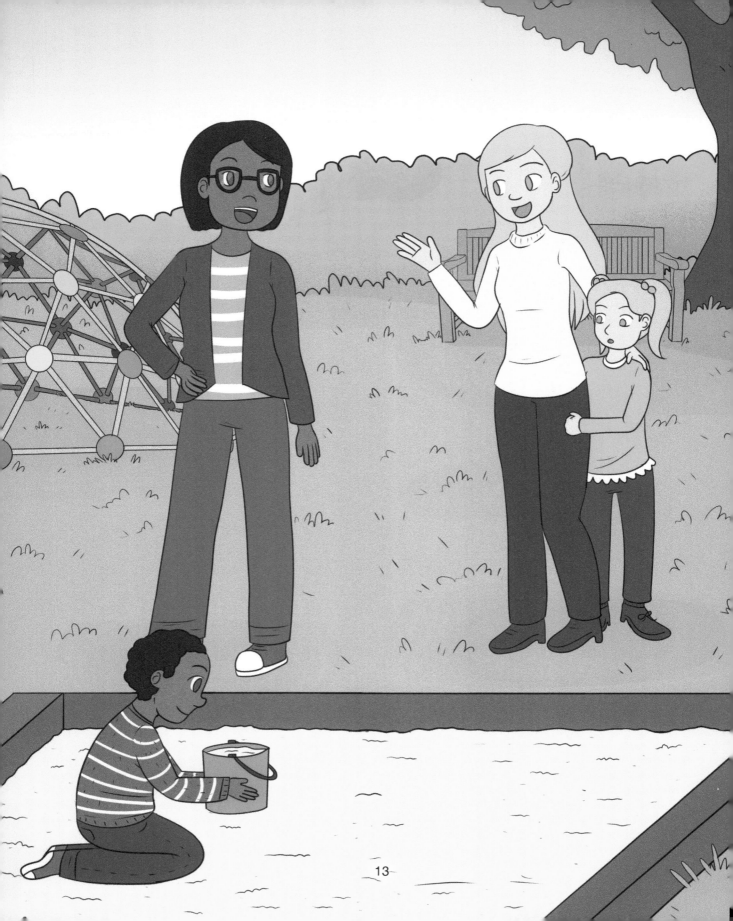

People continued to stare. Jennifer's heart broke as all eyes were on James and Angela. She felt so bad that people were judging and making comments without even knowing James or Angela and the real reason behind why he was upset that day. Angela looked at Jennifer and said, "It's okay. I'm used to this. It happens all the time. The stares, the comments, I'm used to it."

Jennifer's eyes filled up. She hugged Angela and said, "I'm not going to judge." Angela thanked Jennifer, took James by the hand, and walked away. Lilly and Jennifer both silently watched them walk away.

Jennifer and Lilly collected their things and headed home. That night, while Jennifer was putting Lilly to bed, Lilly said, "Mommy, I have some questions about what happened today at the park with the little boy we saw."

"Okay, Lilly," Jennifer said. "Tell me what you want to know."

"Why didn't he want to play with me? Why was he throwing sand and yelling? I don't understand why he was screaming so loudly."

"Well, Lilly," said Jennifer, "James has autism."

"What's autism?" asked Lilly, confused.

"Autism is a disorder where children learn and react differently than most children. There are all several types depending on where you fall on the spectrum. James has the type where he is nonverbal, which means he does not speak."

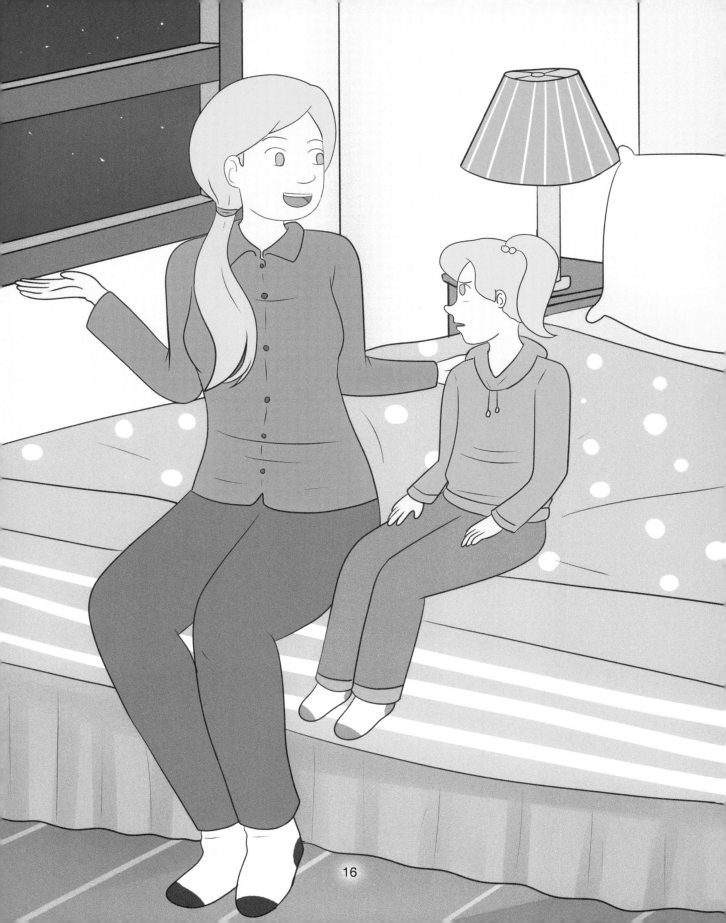

16

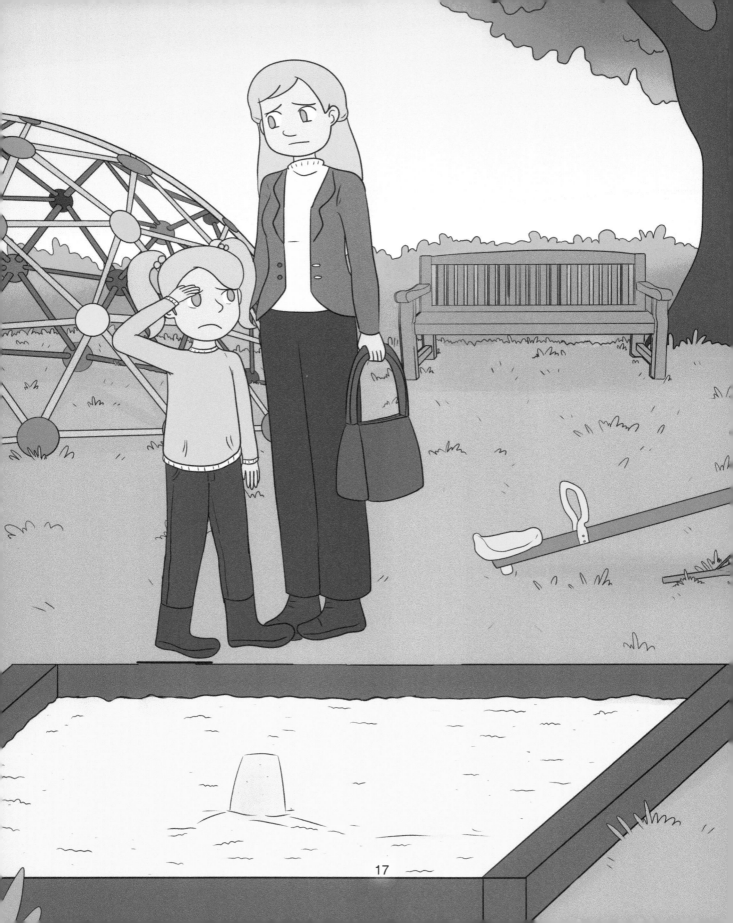

"Oh," said Lilly, "so he's still a kid, just like me, but it seems like he just does things a little different."

"Exactly right," said Jennifer. "Since James cannot tell his mommy why he's upset or what he wants, he will cry or scream to express his feelings to his mommy."

"Can I still be friends with James, Mommy?" Lilly asked.

"Of course, you can," Jennifer said.

The next couple of Saturdays, Jennifer and Lilly packed a lunch bag and went to the park. They waited and waited, and no sign of James or Angela.

"I think we should go," Lilly said. "They're not coming." Just as they were getting ready to leave, Jennifer spotted Angela and James walking down the hill. "James! James!" Lilly cried.

Angela said hello to Jennifer and Lilly.

"Thanks again for the other day," Angela said. "It was nice to have someone not judge and offer help. It made me realize there are still good people in this world."

"No problem at all. You know we come here every Saturday when the weather is nice," Jennifer said.

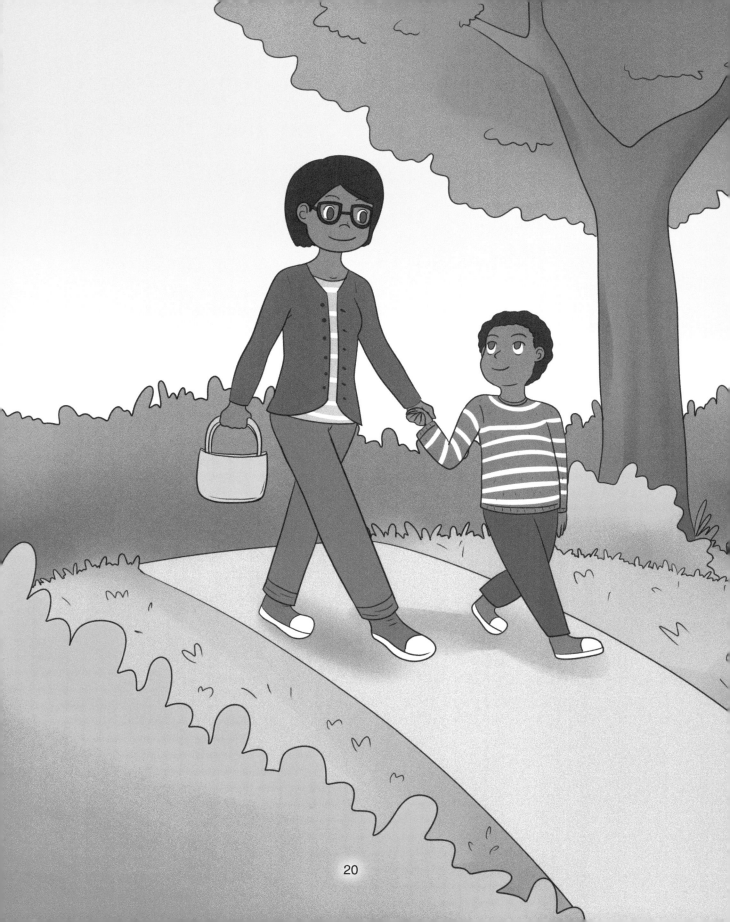

"That's great to know," said Angela. "We will definitely try and meet you here more often when James doesn't have his therapies." Angela and Jennifer looked over. James had a train, and he was playing on the floor with it. Lilly was right beside him, playing with her Barbie doll, trying to pretend she was waiting for a train ride to a magical place.

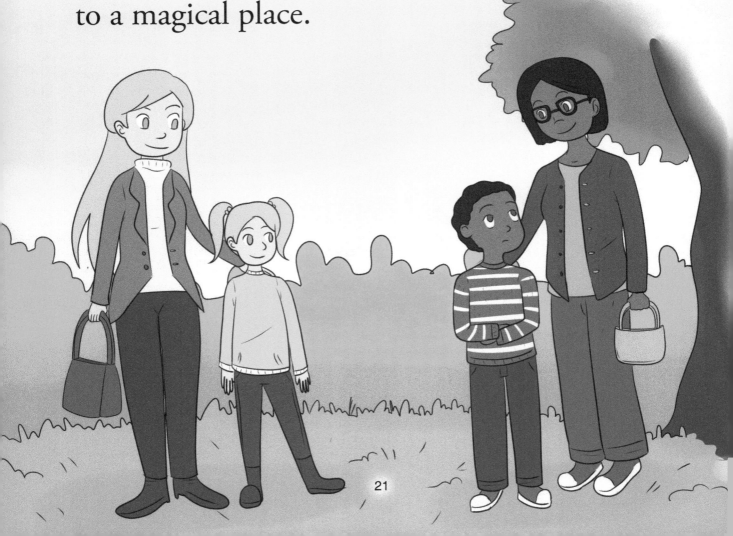

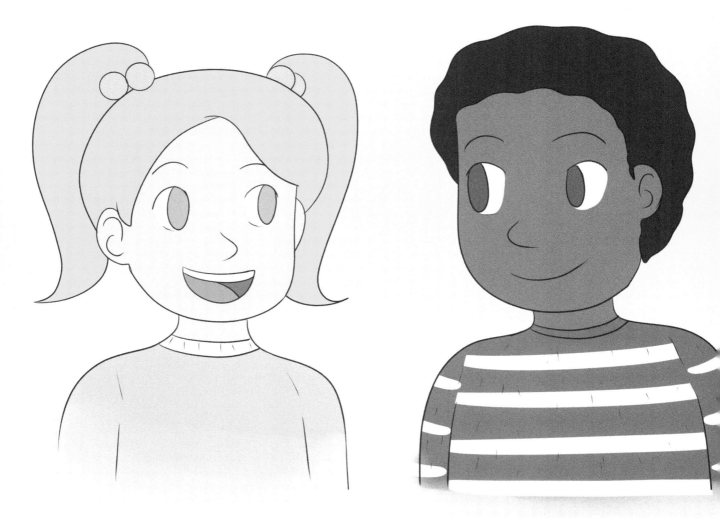

The two played some more before the kids grew tired and went home. On the way home that day, Lilly realized that she could still be friends with James. James just had a unique way of doing things.

Every Saturday they would meet at the park. Angela and Jennifer would drink coffee and catch up on their week while Lilly and James would play side by side. James felt very comfortable with Lilly and would smile big whenever he would see her. Sometimes James would stare at rocks for hours or chase butterflies all day. He loved to do things repeatedly, but he was taking in all the beauty the world had to offer.

Lilly and Jennifer realized that James had a unique way of seeing the world, and his way was beautiful!

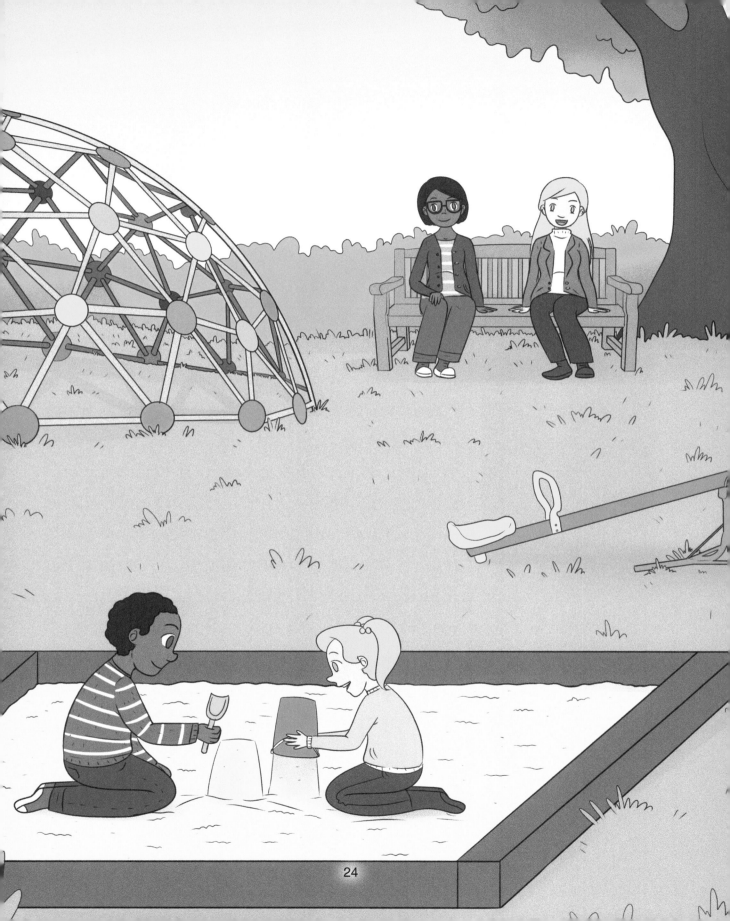

About the Author

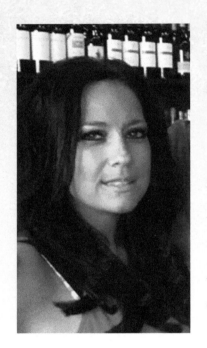

Carmela Fazio-Florio is a special education teacher in Baldwin, New York. She is a wife, and a mother of two beautiful children: Dominick, eight, and Giovanna, five. She grew up in Brentwood, New York, and currently lives in Commack, New York. She has always loved to write as a child and decided to become an author after both years of teaching and having a daughter of her own with delays. Her daughter's delays and experiences have really inspired her to become an author. She felt her books could reach families of children with various disabilities as well as children who would like to learn more about children with special needs. In her free time, she enjoys spending time with her family and friends and traveling. She really hopes these books can reach all children from different walks of life and, of course, teach how being different is not always a negative thing but a beautiful one!